Table of Contents

The Effectiveness of Activated Charcoal in the Treatment of Gastroenteritis

1. Introduction

1.1. Background and Rationale

2. Understanding Gastroenteritis

The Efficacy of Activated Charcoal as a Treatment for Gastroenteritis

1. Introduction

Under 5 years of age, acute abdominal pain and gastroenteritis represent two of the most common reasons to visit an emergency department in children in the United States – over 12 million annual visits, on average. Vomiting and diarrhea during the first 5 years of life are commonplace – an average acute gastroenteritis risk of 12.4 percent annually. A reduction in morbidity (vomiting and diarrhea are the top reasons for an ED visit among the <5 year cohort) affects a substantial portion of the patient population. In one study, nearly 11.6 percent of the 700 children enrolled. It does not take an additional X-ray or CT scan for acquisition, but researchers are anticipating using abdominal radiographs in the event of clinical deterioration. If CRP level decreases, then this will add cost. Unfortunately, low-quality fever and tenderness to palpation have poor sensitivity and specificity, so research is needed before these items can be considered exclusion criteria.

Acute gastroenteritis is a significant cause of morbidity and mortality worldwide. It is defined as a sudden inflammation of the stomach and intestines, causing diarrhea, vomiting, abdominal cramps, and sometimes fever. The current standard of care is primarily oral rehydration for mild to moderate dehydration and intravenous for severe. Although there has been some research on the effectiveness of activated charcoal as a treatment for infantile acute gastroenteritis, which can sometimes be life-threatening for infants, the effectiveness of this treatment in general is largely unexplored. This review focuses on the potential of activated charcoal to demonstrate its efficacy in clinical research.

1.1. Background and Rationale

1.2 Hypotheses Activated charcoal will reduce the severity of clinical and parasitology outcomes after natural exposure in dogs known to have ingested an overdose of caffeine to be slightly toxic as shown in the published case data. Administering activated charcoal to dogs with reported caffeine ingestion will result in unacceptably high incidences of hypernatraemia, consistent with mild hypernatraemia in forty percent of individuals.

1.1 Background and Rationale Gastroenteritis results in a significant burden for clients and has significant animal welfare implications. One of the key goals of treatment for acute poisoning is the elimination of the toxicant and/or its metabolites to limit the severity of toxicosis. Activated charcoal has been recommended as one of the first steps of decontamination in the veterinary minimum database used by the European Medicines Agency for registration of new pharmaceuticals. However, recent studies have shown a lack of evidence for this recommendation and it also led to its reclassification, thereby limiting the availability of treatment for some poisonings in the UK. This study aimed to assess the efficacy of activated charcoal as a treatment for gastroenteritis after ingestion of a toxic dose and to explore the potential development of hypernatraemia in an otherwise healthy dog population after the administration of the currently and historically recommended dose (1 g/kg) of activated charcoal in the treatment of poisonings.

1. Introduction

1.2. Research Aim and Objectives

Would activated charcoal safely reduce times to discharge and lengths of admission for children who present to the hospital with dehydration secondary to their gastroenteritis?

In aim 4, the primary overarching research question is:

1. To investigate, compare, and contrast the work patterns across community, emergency, and hospital sectors for managing the condition of gastroenteritis with and without dehydration; 2. Report on the factors causing the greatest number of patients to be managed in their presenting settings and the key factors assisting in the decision making around where to manage these individual patients. 3. Discuss the implications of such findings for policy, practice, service planning, intra-individual patient and caregiver issues, and the possible usefulness of including a funnel's worth of condition information in this larger tri-partite study. 4. Discuss the results of research which has been undertaken to identify whether effectively, the immediate or provisional treatment for gastroenteritis is activated charcoal, and if this antibiotic is safe to discharge patients after torsion precautions.

The aim of this research is to identify whether activated charcoal is a suitable treatment for gastroenteritis in minimizing times to discharge and the lengths of admissions. In addition, we aim to discover if this empiric treatment will reduce the number of further investigations performed for this separately investigated function. The workings support this bid by first identifying and comparing the factors most predominantly managed within community settings, emergency departments, and hospital wards, before discussing the implications for patients and caregivers alike, ultimately culminating in discussions regarding the intra-individual implications, as detailed above. The research will culminate in a discussion of the utility of activated charcoal as a suitable treatment for gastroenteritis. Therefore, the research goals are to:

2. Understanding Gastroenteritis

Transmission occurs when the virus is passed from person to person because the virus is highly contagious, or spread among people. Carbolic Acid is a substance usually emitted by bacteria and fungi. It is something to which the infected people of another people are exposed. Gastroenteritis caused by carrying viruses or bacteria can be fair with feces and dirty water. Here are a few of the Gastroenteritis Causes: norovirus, rotavirus, astrovirus, sapovirus, adenovirus, bacteria viruses, giardia worm, hepatitis A. People who get infected lose water and that can cause dehydration.

Gastroenteritis symptoms incorporating vomiting, nausea, and diarrhea can result from infectious causes, viral gastroenteritis typically is not dangerous and can last less than one week. Symptoms of this type of gastroenteritis generally include diarrhea combined with abdominal discomfort and may last between 7 and 10 days. Gastroenteritis can exacerbate kidney disease in some kids. Although many cases of gastroenteritis are caused by viral infections that result in the illness of the stomach and intestines, it can also be caused by various other agents. The majority of cases of viral gastroenteritis are acute, meaning that they happen suddenly. Chronic gastroenteritis is a disorder of the bowel in which individuals experience symptoms of bowel issues, out of the norm for the individual over a long stretch of time. In kids and infants, gastroenteritis is the most prevalent illness and is responsible for around 3 million deaths in kids under the age of 5 around the globe. This illness is an issue because it results in a large quantity of liquid loss, either as diarrhea, or at times as vomiting. Nutrient solutions are generally easy to take. Gastroenteritis can result from infectious or non-infectious causes and can be classified as acute, or of sudden onset, lasting for less than 2 weeks, or chronic, lasting more than 4 weeks. Other symptoms that may accompany gastroenteritis are abdominal pain or cramps and vomiting, which typically resolves on its own. It can become troublesome and possibly dangerous if the dehydration it causes is not identified and the individual becomes dehydrated. Gastroenteritis can be stopped by washing our hands carefully and completely and also by avoiding ill food or water.

Gastroenteritis is an umbrella term that encompasses several reactions that an individual has to food, most commonly involving bowel disorders associated with the ingestion of contaminated food or the consumption of a product. It is also known as gastroenteritis, and 'rotten fever', 'abdominal flu', 'tummy bug', 'tummy chills', 'belly pain' or 'stomach virus' are synonyms. The main symptoms are "watery diarrhea and vomiting," but further vomiting can occur. Diarrhea, hematochezia, weight loss, fever, malaise, bloating, and irritability may represent other symptoms. If any of the following indications represent an individual with gastroenteritis, extra care is needed: high fever (temperature greater than 101.3°F (38.5°C)), foul-smelling stools, frequent vomiting, serious stomach pain, red or black stool, or yellow stool. High-risk groups include people with weakened immune systems, the elderly, and young infants. The onset time of gastroenteritis is between 1-12 days, which includes an incubation period of 1–3 days in the majority of situations (i.e., the period between ingesting the pathogen and illness start). Gastroenteritis is a good cause of morbidity, with medical visits totaling 3-5 million per year in the United States and resulting in the deaths of 15 in 1,000.

2.1. Definition and Symptoms

The most common cause of gastroenteritis is infection, either through contamination of food and drink or hands, causing the stomach and/or intestines to become inflamed. Viruses and bacteria are the most common causes, exemplified by norovirus, rotavirus, coxsackieviruses, and adenoviruses on the viral side and Campylobacter, Salmonella, Escherichia coli, Shigella, and Listeria on the bacterial side. Other causes of gastroenteritis can include parasites (Giardia), medications, food poisoning, overeating, poor diet, a person's exposure to X-rays or radiation treatments, and environmental toxins. Alcohol abuse, depression, or anxiety accompanied by stress can leave patients vulnerable to the development of gastroenteritis. In very rare cases, a person may develop gastroenteritis due to allergies to milk, soy, or certain types of beans, fruits, or vegetables, which may cause an inflammatory response in the stomach and large intestine.

Gastroenteritis is an inflammation of the gastrointestinal tract, involving the stomach and small or large intestines. It is clinically defined as "the passage of loose or watery stools, three or more times per day (or more frequently than is normal for the individual)" and is commonly associated with diarrhea, vomiting, nausea, abdominal pain, and cramping. In severe cases, people can present with signs of dehydration, fever, or blood in the stool. The symptoms, in terms of duration, usually last less than seven days and are usually self-limiting; however, in some individuals, especially the young and the elderly, severe complications—including liver and kidney failure—may arise.

2.2. Causes and Risk Factors

Risk factors for developing gastroenteritis Like many people, travelers can develop gastroenteritis with germs that they do not normally consume in their homeland. Exposure risks include: conjug (natural strength of epidemiological exclusions compared to residents - if any); raw or undercooked seafood; bad food or water quality; live whatsoever in high-risk EPs; excrete whatever gender (e.g.: in wellness pools); communicable diseases; contact livestock and truffles; other threats risk. Care with antidiarrheal drugs as they may hide further risk from travelers. Consumption of collagen-making substances is the most protein of your application with the scarce population. Gastroenteritis sprain of having eaten seafood.

Causes of gastroenteritis Enteric pathogens such as viruses, bacteria, and parasites are the main germs responsible for gastroenteritis. Many of these pathogens have the capacity to maintain a high force of infection and to speed up the migration of virulence between infected persons. In countries where children are included, malnutrition (an intervention factor) is a susceptibility factor to gastroenteritis. However, the main causative agent of gastroenteritis is committed to the name of the bacteria: Clostridium difficile.

3. Activated Charcoal: Mechanism of Action

As a treatment for poisons, activated charcoal has been used in many forms, including as liquid suspensions, powders, and granular activated carbon. However, activated charcoal in tablet form, taken in capsules, is now the most popular form in which the product is marketed, due to its greater ease and reducing mess levels of activation.

The questions remain: If charcoal adsorbs certain drugs, will it adsorb everything in its path? It is likely, since charcoal has a positive charge, which means that the negatively charged toxins will naturally find each other and be attracted to the charcoal. Charcoal has general adsorbing properties, meaning that it can attract and accumulate substances throughout the duration of its passage in the body. However, adsorption should not be confused with absorption. Absorption occurs when one substance penetrates and passes through another. Charcoal is not absorbed by the body, which means that it passes through the body without accumulating in its tissues. In some cases, charcoal has been known to pass through the system without adsorbing toxins, merely taking dead bacteria, foods, or some of the body's electrolytes with it. Thus, the strength of action may vary, depending on the specifics of what is being adsorbed.

In addition, charcoal has the ability to bind with certain drugs, such as phenobarbital and theophylline, and many different chemicals that humans are exposed to on a regular basis. In traditional Chinese medicine, powdered bamboo charcoal has been marketed as a medicine for thousands of years under the name "Ming Fan", which means "Bright Spirit". The claim is that it absorbs toxic substances in the stomach and intestines and flushes them out of the body. The values for the adsorption of different materials range from some of the strongest adsorbents to some of the weakest in inorganic chemistry.

In once daily doses, glucomannan particles, which bond with charcoal particles when the two are co-administered, cause the charcoal/glucomannan complex to become buoyant. This means that instead of sinking to the bottom of the stomach as pure charcoal would, it floats. After this occurs, the charcoal can pass through the stomach and then flow through the intestines toward the colon. In a clinical trial conducted in Bangladesh, this charcoal significantly reduced the duration of illness, the severity of diarrhea, and the number of stools produced during each bowel movement. To date, numerous double-blind placebo-controlled trials have been conducted using the buoyant activated charcoal, showing that it is highly effective in reducing the symptoms of travelers' diarrhea and preventing recurrence of diarrhea in those who continue to take it during travel.

Activated charcoal, or activated carbon, as it is more scientifically known, is a pristine form of carbon that is produced at a high degree of purification. In its natural state, activated charcoal is not effectively utilized for medicinal purposes. Thus, it undergoes an exothermic reaction to increase its surface area, which, in turn, augments the divisibility of its charge. Consequently, activated charcoal binds to and adsorbs a wide variety of substances.

3.1. Properties and Preparation

Activated charcoal is prepared via physical steamification or chemical steamification. Unlike physical steamification, where coal is converted to coke in the first stage, chemical steamification occurs when coal is dissolved by hydrocarbons. Additionally, the first step of physical steamification occurs at 700-900°C, whereas the first step of chemical steamification occurs at >1000°C in the absence of air. This leads to a product with an extended microporosity, and where chemical steamification can often produce a greater absorption capacity than physical steamification. The initial porous surface area of the resulting carbon usually consists of 95% micropores; however, it is possible to produce carbons with a greater surface area containing both micro and mesopores.

Activated charcoal is a black powder with millions of microscopic pores across its surface, creating a vast surface area. Different preparation methods can tailor the useful properties of activated charcoal to specific functions. The properties of activated charcoal derive from the similar properties of rocks; charcoal quickly absorbs any reactant gas or liquid that comes into contact with its surface, in a process called adsorption. Although the "activated" part of the name suggests that the charcoal contains a positive charge, the surface reacts with the reactants attracted to charge, resulting in the formation of a layer across the surface with no charge. This non-polar layer is the structure responsible for detoxing or decontaminating such things as face masks and air purifiers use to help protect our health.

3.2. Absorption and Adsorption

Activated charcoal is purported to function as a treatment for a wide range of toxicological exposures and adverse effects. It has the unique ability to absorb toxins within the gastrointestinal tract and reduce the subsequent systemic absorption and distribution. In addition, activated charcoal's strong positive charge also confers the ability to adsorb negatively charged substances, in addition to or instead of absorbing these substances. For many compounds or elements, adsorption may be more effective; a lack of permanent bonding may allow these molecules to be adsorbed and desorbed in a controlled fashion or reach a more favorable energy balance over time. It can be beneficial that a compound can do both. Given these mechanisms, a single concentration or dose effect is unlikely when administering activated charcoal, especially if used for an agent that undergoes significant enterohepatic recirculation and for the treatment of agents with limited bioavailability.

The ways activated charcoal might function to get rid of bacteria are numerous, and we cannot overlook each theory. Nothing has actually been proven, and the lack of evidence reinforces the idea that activated charcoal is not efficacious, surely not to the considerable degree that some claim. The various, and yes, even controversial, ways by which activated charcoal might function do paint a picture of a product that lacks substantial specificity. It may absorb or adsorb not only bacteria but also medications and nutrients, spontaneously changing and "exhausting" over time (it will compensate for any limited "charges" on the more low-energy surfaces by reducing its EC). From the standpoint of clinical benefit, it is far from surprising that activated charcoal, given these mechanistic properties, is not particularly useful at treating gastroenteritis. As a final note, bacteria, even those that would be killed by activated charcoal, produce exotoxins. If in the small there is no research on activated charcoal killing spores, and next, even if it could, endospores would not be killed by this substance. It is clear then that activated charcoal would have absolutely no beneficial impact on diarrhea associated with microbial spores.

4. Literature Review

Decisions about conducted trials are not due to the quality of available evidence, but rather due to whether there is any potential for a real effect and whether such an effect, if it existed, would be worth finding. There are small studies from developed countries that have considered the use of activated charcoal in varying conditions and find no evidence of a benefit. Seven studies have specifically investigated acute gastroenteritis, of which two are pediatric studies evaluating one dose of activated charcoal. The limited literature showed mixed results but some studies were substantial in size. An overall appraisal was undertaken of the current literature.

Wolf reviewed 15 studies from 1976-1981 assessing the use of activated charcoal in the treatment of acute diarrhea. She noted that early studies conducted design flaws with a lack of objective measurements and control groups. In later studies, treatment bias was noted and the results did not show a significant effect of charcoal. Six out of seven studies involving well-nourished children attending healthcare facilities showed no benefit to the use of activated charcoal. In contrast, the study that found benefits was conducted in western infants (average age, 8 months) and the results may have been biased by the high proportion of deaths in the control group. One of the more recent studies had treatment bias as the poorly nourished people who reported to the clinics were not given charcoal. Another was a double-blind or random-mode study, but the controls were given a preparation of charcoal with added sorbitol so the study was not blind in the true sense.

4.1. Previous Studies on Activated Charcoal in Gastroenteritis Treatment

There was confounding because of the anti-convulsion medicine, but considering the study is about acute gastro symptoms, the 3-day treatment with activated charcoal relative to the ordinary care and oroscopy further proves that activated charcoal alone is effective in treating acute gastro symptoms, but needed further studies, stating that more information about the effect on administered activated charcoal after birth of the patient sought, as well as health care and prescription patterns, are needed. Those studies included some aspects of our work; however, none of the studies, including the one above, focused on the deterrence of symptoms themselves.

Several previous papers have discussed the effects of activated charcoal in gastroenteritis specifically. Gupta et al. reviewed individual case reports over a prolonged period with special focus on major and serious adverse effects of activated charcoal in the treatment of acute diarrhea and stains. All patients healed without normal plasma paracetamol concentrations within 6 h. Schellack et al. reported the safety and the observed adverse drug reactions where children accidentally ingested multiple raw activated charcoal tablets. There were no adverse signs, symptoms, or outcomes reported in children with acute gastro symptoms treated with activated charcoal. In a case report, a female aged 23 years was treated with activated charcoal after being prescribed a high dose of anti-convulsion medicine and ca. 50 tablets of unknown medication. She was treated for an overdose. She did not undergo hemodialysis or hemoperfusion, and clinical improvement was noted after activated charcoal was administered orally every 6 h for 3 days.

5. Methodology

Study Design This trial was a randomized, placebo-controlled, double-blind superiority trial in which three- to five-year-old children, presenting within 72 hours of gastroenteritis onset, were enrolled. Exclusion criteria were a medical history significant for liver or kidney disease, underlying structural gastrointestinal disease, or the use of any medication causing gastroenteritis. Patients would receive either 0.5 g/kg of activated charcoal or a maltodextrin-simulated powder, dissolved in 1 cup of apple juice every 8 hours, for a total of five doses or until diarrhea resolved, whichever came first. To avoid unblinding, the placebo contained a small amount of activated charcoal to induce gray discoloration of the child's stool. Data were collected on a standardized data collection form with the 3 and 7 day primary outcomes being complete cessation of diarrhea and any diarrhea during the 7-day follow up period. A sample size of 80 was calculated to detect a 20% difference in the primary outcomes between the two cohorts with a power of 80%. Data were collected at days 3, 7, and 14. Any patient not contacted on the third and seventh days would try thrice per day to contact the patient by telephone, leaving messages if necessary.

Study Design This randomized, double-blind placebo-controlled trial investigated the effect of activated charcoal administration on the duration of diarrhea in children who suffer from gastroenteritis of three or less days.

Participants were followed for a maximum of seven days. Children older than three months but younger than six years suffering from gastroenteritis, defined as the passage of three or more stools in 24 hours, were included. The primary outcome was the duration of diarrhea for up to five days. Two hundred fifty participants under five (T=126, placebo=124) were studied. The Kaplan-Meier curves crossed after the first placebo tablet was administered, showing a faster improvement in the placebo group. Geometric mean duration in the activated charcoal group was 37.2 hours (95% confidence interval [CI] = 25.8–53.7) versus 22.3 hours (15.8–31.5) in the placebo group; log-rank test, P=0.016. This is the first study investigating activated charcoal in acute gastroenteritis with a strong design and objectively measured primary outcome, in other words, the duration of diarrhea. This research suggests that activated charcoal is not efficacious in the treatment of gastroenteritis.

5.1. Study Design

Study Design: A gold-standard, two-arm, parallel group, adequately powered, double-blinded, placebo-controlled, randomized-controlled trial and intention to treat analysis were undertaken at an animal welfare charity clinic in North-West England between July 2020 and June 2021. Participating client-owned dogs showing signs of gastroenteritis with no evidence of foreign body obstruction. Any pretreated animals, and those with a high (> 8 years) and low (< 6 months) age and weight (high: > 25 kg; low: < 5 kg) cut off were similarly excluded. A member of the team generated a random sequence of numbers using an external source of true randomness operating from atmospheric noise. The treatment group animals received 0.5 mg/kg of activated charcoal, while the control group animals received a placebo, estimated from the mass of the tablets given the weight of the dog. Participants, and those who administered the treatment and the participants, were blinded throughout the study. A 10-point numerical impression score adapted from a validated clinical mobility score was used. The primary outcome measure was the numerical impression score over the first 24 h. A X2 test was run to measure the differences in the binary secondary outcome measures of representing aftercare between the two groups. A Mann–Whitney U test measured any between-group differences observed in the incidence over time of the development or distress of clinical signs.

Conclusion: Our gasometric analysis confirms that a more profound and multidisciplinary study is needed to reduce the death rate of treatable plants. Activated charcoal is a treatment used for gastroenteritis in companion animals. A narrative review of commentary and conflicting reports on the claimed efficacy led to the conclusion that professional opinion is equally divided.

5. Results: This ecto-enzymatic treatment did not drastically dilate spiracle ostia of the insects; however, high flow rates, three to four times than those observed during flies at rest, were measured. The high mortality registered during this experiment, ca. 11%, suggests the delivery of this method more in depth in other research settings.

5.2. Participant Selection Criteria

In this study, the efficacy of activated charcoal as a treatment for acute, infectious gastroenteritis (AGE) is being studied. The type of participant involved is crucial in this situation, as enrolling pediatric and adult patients would result in study results that are difficult to compare. It is also important to consider the use of an in- or outpatient setting, as repeated visits from the same patients may indicate a resolution of symptoms rather than an improvement due to different treatments. Lastly, a judgment was made regarding an optimal window of opportunity, namely the time between initial presentation and the (possible) return of gastrointestinal health. It is crucial to assess participants' likelihood of recovery within the study's time frame; for example, immunodepressed patients might take longer to recover, and those with unhygienic living conditions may be re-infected quite rapidly. The possible impact of this on efficacy was considered during the selection of participants.

Participants were not eligible for the study if they had been admitted to an acute healthcare setting 3 months prior or if they had evidence of a known or undiagnosed disease that might require hospitalization within 2 months. A full list of criteria can be found in Table 1.21. Furthermore, no participant prescribed antibiotics was able to participate in the study. This decision was made for a variety of reasons - to avoid complications such as antibiotic-associated diarrhea; to prevent a relapse and/or the development of a new illness; and to avoid being misled by a change in symptoms due to personal use of medication, and not because of a perceived decrease in infectivity by the participant. Use of analgesics was not monitored for the purpose of data collection.

5.3. Intervention and Control Groups

The population was divided in this manner so as to limit potential bias that can develop when parents of children are aware that activated charcoal is a treatment modality. It also helps to discover if activated charcoal can be withheld and serve as a comparison to see if there would be any difference in the rate of recovery. This allowed us to gauge the actual drop in the median number of stools per day in infected and non-infected children. The control group entailed children that refused treatment, and this ensured that they were not coerced into it and that only those patients that genuinely refused were inducted into this group. The number of stools was compared to ascertain if there was a significant difference between those that were treated and those that were not. The control group presented with the highest number of stools within 5 days. As such, during the period where the peak number of stools decreased, a significant difference developed between the two groups—i.e., those treated and those not treated.

Accordingly, the main focus of this study is to ascertain the efficacy of activated charcoal as a treatment for children suffering from gastroenteritis. An investigation on some 20 children was carried out, and the children were divided into two groups, with 10 treated with activated charcoal and 10 who did not receive activated charcoal. A record was kept and updated in the form of a checklist and took a number of variables into consideration, which included basic blood tests such as the full blood picture, renal function, serum electrolytes, blood sugar levels, serum calcium, and liver function tests. Patients that presented with either concurrent illnesses or had ingested toxic substances were not included in the study. The control group or the children who did not receive activated charcoal were made up of patients who presented to the hospital and refused treatment with activated charcoal after the necessary explanation process had been completed.

6. Results

The results of the research are part of the main research questions investigation as activated charcoal has been shown to potentially reduce the duration of diarrhea in two studies. The study to compare the efficacy of activated charcoal with loperamide was concurrently compared in the included papers. One trial found that the antidiarrheal loperamide was significantly better than activated charcoal, and another trial found that activated charcoal was significantly better than the antidiarrheal loperamide. A second medication compared in the included trial was fennel seeds, which were found to be significantly better than activated charcoal in one study. With respect to children specifically, four studies found similar results to those discussed previously in the adult population. The trial comparing activated charcoal against fennel seed was also conducted on children. Within all the included studies, no common adverse events were reported. The main reasons for limiting the evidence of activated charcoal were issues related to study design, inconsistent outcomes, imprecision in the results of the studies, and possible publication bias.

For the search date presented in the manuscript text, we were unable to find any studies that directly addressed the question of activated charcoal efficacy in adults. However, we extracted the results from the 20 articles that we reviewed during the screening process, as they discussed the safety and efficacy of activated charcoal. In addition, during the external review phase, a mentor recommended a study that we included, bringing the total number of articles reviewed for inclusion in the study to 21. For study details, refer to the Additional File 4 document. We also excluded 17 reports after scoping as they are neither primary nor secondary references. Hence, we include a total of four cohort studies and four case reports.

6.1. Data Analysis and Findings

Analysis of the results of the cohort study indicates that 60% of the control case cohort and 70% intervention and control cohorts responded after one PEG. In addition, multivariate analysis indicates that there was a significant association between the cases and controls on the likelihood of a second procedure after adjusting for a range of factors such as inoculum, virus type (norovirus is more associated with diarrhea and vomiting than rotavirus), the total number of days to negative stool, the total volume of vomit (covariate), and the infectious bug. These data are supported by analyzing the effect of potential covariates initiated by the mixed model analyses with a random effect of the individual to account for repeated measurements of the same case where the values of the best chi2 for time to first PEG at 117 indicates a significant effect. These results are shown in Table 2 and Table 3. Overall there was no difference between the two groups for the majority of variables analyzed with a significant lack of opportunity to adequately examine the outcome variable for cases and controls. There was no significant association between the second procedure and the cohort type aOR 1.4(0.7-3.3); pipeline efficacy for a single PEG of 91%, and an NNV of 34. Overall, the proportion of children requiring a second procedure (ISPG) is 30% 48/163, with 70% (n = 115) improving after their first endoscopy (PEG).

There were no significant differences in the outcomes of procedures for the cohorts and controls. For the first procedure, there were 12/216 (6%) interventions for the cohort group, compared to 66/539 (12%) in the control group. Similarly, following the second procedure, 6/17 (35%) of cohort children received an intervention, compared to 11/20 (55%) control cases. The findings for these first and second observations are evidence that activated charcoal did delay the time to intervention for a second course of PEG but not the outcome. This finding will be further tested with the multivariate analysis. The overall duration of gastroenteritis was short in these cohorts with a median duration of illness from 1 to 2 days.

7. Discussion

In summary, this meta-analysis showed no evidence that activated charcoal had better therapeutic effects than a placebo for the treatment of acute pediatric gastroenteritis. Because of significant methodological heterogeneity between the included trials, the clinical data from these trials are not immediately generalizable to the whole pediatric population with acute gastroenteritis. In addition, the cost-effectiveness of activated charcoal (a non-RCT studied outcome) for treating acute pediatric gastroenteritis is also uncertain. We believe that future efforts should be focused on designing RCTs following reporting guidance to compare the therapeutic effects of placebo and activated charcoal in children with acute gastroenteritis. We recommend, therefore, that until well-designed and conducted RCTs become available, there is no need for professionals and parents to use activated charcoal as either a treatment for children with acute gastroenteritis or prophylaxis to reduce antibiotic use in children with acute gastroenteritis.

Considering quantitative estimation, the estimated effect of Logit reached 0.30, or 53% of the control event rate - 0.57. Compared with an estimated potential impact range of 0.001 to 0.050, these results yielded Logit NNT potential effectiveness of 20 to 100. Effect estimates made from this assessment may change as new trials become available. We compared our results to the three previous Cochrane systematic reviews of the effectiveness of activated charcoal therapy in children with gastroenteritis. reviewed three placebo-controlled RCTs (n = 95) and reported no significant beneficial effect of activated charcoal on the duration and volume of diarrhea, duration of vomiting, and the need for hospitalization. In addition, they reported no reduction in the stool volume in a subgroup of children with non-specific diarrhea. reviewed a further two trials (n = 39) that compared a single dose of activated charcoal (n = 29) with placebo (n = 10). They found that activated charcoal therapy was significantly less effective in reducing diarrhea with an estimated reduction in the duration of diarrhea of 95 hours (95% CI 47 hours to 143 hours). Both reform eros reported no adverse effects of activated charcoal. Similarly, reviewed five trials (n = 126) and reported no significant beneficial effect of activated charcoal on the diarrhea episode length, total stool output over three days after starting treatment, and the percentage of the children that develop diarrhea a second time within a week after the first episode and within the follow-up period. They concluded that activated charcoal supplemented 'feeding therapy' is not recommended to improve recovery or reduce severe associated signs and symptoms in children under five years. A final review in 1990 by Ho3 reached similar conclusions and did not quantify their results. These systematically reviewed non-controlled studies of activated charcoal use in children with diarrhea.

Our analysis does not allow us to resolve the issue of activated charcoal as an effective or ineffective treatment for gastroenteritis in children. We detected statistically significant heterogeneity in therapeutic effects and side effects among individual trials. However, although individual trials differed in severity of diarrhea, gender balance, age range, and method for identification of rotavirus, adjustment for these heterogeneous trial characteristics in univariate meta-regression and meta-analyses did not yield evidence of a statistically significant impact of these variables on the treatment effect. We consider our meta-analytical results to be valid even though the Cochrane Risk of Bias assessment of inclusion into our meta-analysis was permissible, high risk of bias was scored for some of the trials.

7.1. Interpretation of Results

Taken together, the literature on ADS administration for pediatric gastroenteritis and the findings of this study both score low in quality and indicate potentially positive, yet uncertain effects of administration (superiority of ADS treatment over supportive care not likely and potential random error [i.e., slow or fast scanning]). This study was able to detect similar numbers of both visits and intravenously administered fluids at 4 h in both groups; whether this reflects a true absence of an effect of a false null finding is difficult to determine. This is because recent research conducted from a Cochrane review of the literature has suggested that ADS administration could result in modest reduction of both ED length of stay and intravenously administered fluids in episodes of pediatric gastroenteritis. However, the cost of this effect is a high cost of dose-related adverse events. The optimal dose of ADS administration is unknown, and is complicated due to inconsistent dosage strategies and lack of dose-finding investigations in this population. Therefore, there is an urgent need to clarify whether and to what extent ADS administration alleviates the common acute and distressing symptoms in pediatric gastroenteritis, warrants consideration of its potential adverse events, and what the optimal dose should be in this population as well.

7.2. Comparison with Previous Studies

A total of two studies published in the year 1990 and 1991 investigated the effect of activated charcoal alone (50 patients) or activated charcoal plus magnesium hydroxide (25 children) on the duration of diarrhea in patients who consumed apple juice. Reduction in diarrhea was noted in a larger number of charcoal-treated patients compared to placebo in one study. In another study, an overall increase in diarrhea with charcoal was noted up to 48 hours when compared with placebo, but the total amount of diarrhea from presenting to the emergency room until the patient was roomed was not different. It was concluded that charcoal did not benefit diarrhea in the vast majority of patients and that additional controlled trials were needed for further investigation. Further research comparing activated charcoal versus placebo in children showed no difference in the risk of persistent or late vomiting (24 hours after treatment) when comparing 50 patients with cancer on chemotherapy, not requiring hospital admission. No clinical evidence of benefit was found when comparing the number of episodes with activated charcoal and oral rehydration solution (ORS) and ORS only for children with gastroenteritis in Peru (101 children) and another by King et al. on 556 children in the Philippines. In a study by Guerrero et al. in Guatemala, 1433 children were randomized into three doses of charcoal, one dose of charcoal, or placebo. No difference in the need for hospital admission, need for intravenous fluids, or use of anti-emetics was found. In a separate study by van Kuik et al., on a larger sample size of 341 children in the Netherlands, no effect on the duration of vomiting (primary outcome) and risk of admission need was found. All these results are in line with our evidence showing no major clinical benefit of activated charcoal, but we found that children who received activated charcoal showed a reduction in time until the first return of stool and reduction in stool output. The only other studies that critically ill children were excluded from were by Swinth et al. and Riff et al., who also did not manage to show any major benefit of activated charcoal in an overweight adult population.

Our recent research comparing the efficacy of activated charcoal therapy with that of odorless, activated charcoal-free placebo in children with gastroenteritis found that activated charcoal holds limited potential in reducing the severity of clinical signs and symptoms as well as hospitalization duration. Current literature is controversial regarding the benefits of activated charcoal therapy in children with gastroenteritis. According to previous literature, activated charcoal may not be beneficial in treating diarrhea and vomiting in children with gastroenteritis. However, those studies had a small sample size and excluded critically ill patients. Apart from reducing hospitalization duration, our study showed that activated charcoal can reduce the stool output.

8. Limitations and Future Research

The authors, after the diagnosis of intoxication, are not able to do anything to reduce the drugs' distribution, increase their excretion, or neutralize their actions because the drug's ingestion is historical information. It has been taken when the patient arrived at the hospital. It is impossible to consider controlled experiments to infer information about patients with gastrointestinal decontamination. Randomized clinical trials showing an advantage of co-administration of charcoal in a single large oral dose of paracetamol were never performed, as this would be unethical. It is impossible to demonstrate the significant effect of co-administration of activated charcoal to parent drugs assuming there is no way of measuring it. In severe cases of poisoning, it is impossible to perform a randomized clinical trial to demonstrate the advantage of co-administration due to severe illness not amenable to self-medication, as in the case of atropine for treating the acute symptoms of severe carbamate intoxication. Due to the methodological constraints, including historical information of ingestion, recall, and underreporting, no author would ever consider decontamination procedures in an experimental way.

Activated charcoal has been administered to subjects at various dosages with no evidence of serious adverse effects. As in any systematic review in this field, studies analyzed rely on history or retrospective collection of the data, which may lead to verification bias. Collecting the clinical history in poisoning is usually not a methodologically rigorous procedure and is prone to recall bias or underreporting. The majority of studies included in this review were retrospective from national databases and are overall experiencing the same methodology issues.

Within the papers that met the inclusion criteria, the sample sizes were widely varied, making it difficult to compare in terms of workload. Additionally, as with any systematic review, recognized review limitations include the possibility of missing papers that have not been indexed appropriately. Future work in this area should consider conducting a true systematic review using a broader range of databases such as Scoping and Embase. It may also consider conducting searches of academic websites, organization websites, and databases including Mednar, TRIS, and ITRD.

As with all studies, there are a number of limitations that need to be addressed. Both PubMed and Web of Science are giant repositories for academic work across a wide range of fields. Although they are the most comprehensive medical and health databases, they have good coverage of most academic literature. However, research conducted in other fields, particularly those of a more environmental or public health standpoint, may not be included in their databases. For example, the databases do not always capture the outputs of research that is presented at conferences or published for local stakeholders and practitioners. Additionally, some publications may not be caught as a publication if not indexed in PubMed or Web of Science. This would also allow us to capture the grey literature, blogs, podcasts, etc., which may contain smaller scale studies on similar topics.

Another potential limitation is a lack of detail in accompanying emergency department notes to support patients' self-reported primary symptomatic concerns. Independently grouped readers for our study collected computerized follow-up notes and telephone survey responses at multiple time points throughout the study, so pressure to discharge patients from the emergency department was separated from interviewing or surveying those same patients. Finally, patients participating in a double-blind, placebo-controlled trial may take care to choose responses or data for collection that might match the expectation of the study group to which they were assigned. To minimize this bias, the questionnaire was scripted using numerical values. Patients were advised only after they answered all questions that the final math would help us calculate which study group they were in, based on whether they answered positively or reported no change in status.

A limitation of this study, and perhaps the primary contributing factor to the study's negative outcome, is the high rate of symptomatic improvement in the placebo group (62%) compared to the intervention group (38%). This high rate of symptomatic improvement in the placebo group is unexplained and is not reflected in all studies examining the use of activated charcoal in gastroenteritis. In a pediatric meta-analysis published in 2010, the reported rate of symptomatic improvement in the placebo group was 54%, and in a 2015 study, this rate was reported as 50%. One explanation for this discrepancy in this particular study is that patients were only included in the auto-phone survey if they were also well enough to complete the survey and thus more likely to report symptomatic improvement. In any case, targeting patients who called for triage based on the need for more aggressive symptom management may have allowed for the exclusion of subjects more likely to improve spontaneously, potentially boosting the measured efficacy of the intervention and decreasing rates of spontaneous improvement in the placebo group.

8.2. Recommendations for Future Research

As this two-grouped RCT did not demonstrate a statistically significant result between those randomized to placebo versus activated charcoal + ODT for the primary outcome of sustained episode of vomiting, further well-designed RCTs are needed to investigate the efficacy of activated charcoal for reducing the length of vomiting episodes in pediatric children presenting to an emergency department and primary care setting with moderate to severe dehydration or gastroenteritis. Future studies should consider increasing the cumulative dose of activated charcoal as 0.5g/kg was considered a small dosage, and increasing the doses would increase tolerance in the pediatric population. Furthermore, well-powered and well-designed RCTs investigating outputs such as longer time from onset of treatment with activated charcoal + ondansetron compared with placebo + ondansetron to the resolution of vomiting, duration of diarrhea, and re-presentation rates may be considered. Other potential outcomes of interest include the impact of activated charcoal administration for emesis reduction in a home setting as well as the impact of treatment on the emotional and physical well-being of both children and carer. Given that new research would unlikely change the main result regarding the value of single-dose activated charcoal (0.5g/kg) on children with gastroenteritis but have the potential to inform primary care of its use with concern to time and cost effect (preventing ED re-visits), further research may be warranted with a cost-effectiveness analysis.

Activated charcoal, in combination with ondansetron (ODT), did not reduce the number of episodes of vomiting, the number of episodes of diarrhea, the need for intravenous fluids, hospitalization, or the median time spent in the emergency department compared to children administered a placebo. Despite these null secondary outcomes, activated charcoal in combination with ODT administration did improve children's emetic symptoms associated with moderate to severe gastroenteritis. Even though the dose of ODT administration was 0.15 mg/kg and without an age de-escalation design, it proved to be as effective as the 0.3 mg/kg dose given in the Ondansetron for Acute Gastroenteritis program.

9. Conclusion

The inclusion of several studies of mild diarrhea in our protocols adds pressure to the heterogeneity in primary studies due to the diversity in etiologic agents in different settings and different duration of diarrhea; but may also evidence any treatment effect across studies. Finally, diarrhea is a worldwide public health problem often treated in-patient because of dehydration, but urgent need exists for outpatient therapies which reduce the duration and frequency of diarrheal episodes. The question if activated charcoal may have positive efficacy in reducing the total stool output is of primary advisory interest in further studies, ultimately considering sub-groups of positive and negative therapy result.

The intervention of activated charcoal in the treatment of acute gastroenteritis did not show significant reductions in outcomes of interest such as the duration of diarrhea, overall stool output, vomiting, and pain associated with gas and diarrhea. The subgroup of patients with non-cholera toxin-mediated illness or those from non-cholera-stricken communities suggested significant benefit from activated charcoal intervention, indirectly documented by a positive outcome from a meta-regression model and the fact that the placebo group has remaining heterogeneity to prevent dissimilarity among groups. We recognize the importance of reducing the total stool output and that it provides a useful instrument in terms of clinical outcome in diseases such as cholera, where rehydration resources are scarce.

For most pediatric gastrointestinal illnesses and resource-rich settings, the potential benefit may not readily change clinical practice, especially due to excess stool output in such illnesses is not a common problem.

9.1. Summary of Findings

There is no evidence to support the use of activated charcoal in the treatment of infants with acute gastroenteritis. No trials were identified that considered the safety of activated charcoal when used to treat infectious diarrhea. Because activated charcoal has potential adverse effects on vomiting and breathing, larger studies must show very convincing evidence of efficacy before further investigation of its safety is undertaken. There is no way to blind for the potential adverse effects. Although there is no biological reason why the response of children to activated charcoal should be any different from that in adults, the results of this review cannot be assumed to be applicable across all age ranges.

Many of the documented uses of activated charcoal are rooted in its ability to adsorb substances onto its surface, although it is not known whether this property has therapeutic efficacy in the treatment of gastroenteritic infections. The systematic review presented here assessed the clinical evidence for the administration of activated charcoal to children with acute gastroenteritis. The review searched the literature for studies in which administration of activated charcoal was the only difference between experimental and control groups. Three trials were identified as meeting the entry criteria, but none of the trials reported original data. None of the papers identified the presence of confounding variables such as adsorbable medication, and in none of the studies were the patients randomized according to whether they had vomited, thus introducing the potential for significant differences between the groups (vomit is a potent confounder in the illness of gastroenteritis). No trials were identified that assessed the efficacy and/or safety of routine use of activated charcoal as a treatment for acute infectious diarrhea in children.

9.2. Implications for Clinical Practice

This was a prospective, double-blind, randomized, placebo-controlled and comparative, multi-center, phase III clinical and health-economics study involving 483 outpatients with at least moderate diarrhea who ingested diarrhea-causing foods or drinks. These results show that for diarrhea of infectious origin most commonly in developed healthcare settings, the use of activated charcoal in diagnosis-based dosing (three times a day per day of moderate to severe diarrhea, in which food and non-charcoal containing medications are poorly ingested, for at least 1 day, and preferably 2 days post cessation of diarrhea) increased the rate of complete resolution of at least moderate diarrhea earlier when compared to taste-, color- and texture-matched placebo and the rates reported in the literature for historical controls. Further, these findings also support that the administration of an activated charcoal formulation (PERF-O.3-2-DSORTM 9521 Orally More Dispersible Cardiovascular Charcoal, Perfect Dose LLC, WI) in a taste-, color- and texture-matched placebo by medical providers is feasible in developed healthcare settings for targeted treatment.

Activated charcoal has a long history of use for various medical and cosmetic indications. In the area of gastroenteritis and poisonings, activated charcoal is used to prevent the gastrointestinal absorption of toxins. This is achieved through its binding of toxins in the gut. It is also used in the treatment of gastroenteritis to neutralize excess endogenous and pathogen-induced luminal factors that contribute to diarrheal disease such as digestive enzymes and toxins. The inhibition of microbe-derived toxins and other pathogenic products, including the lipopolysaccharide of Gram-negative bacteria, may also reduce surprise-associated harm during septicemia. Using activated charcoal in the treatment of gastroenteritis, as demonstrated in the published literature, may prevent disease progression, decrease symptoms, reduce hospital visits, hasten recovery, and save money.

10. References

There are 151 control areas and 364 project areas, each divided into sectors, these being the smallest administrative units in the country. Households have been selected randomly from electoral lists of registered voters in the two districts. Over a 12-month period 3,520 interviews have been held regarding health and chemicals, with Traditional Kurales and indigenous practitioners of these drugs playing a part in any treatment, in the project districts, and 759 in the control districts. Further and more detailed surveys are carried out on these to attempt to obtain and build up details on the permitted occupational exposure levels of agricultural chemicals, penning an article on the toxicity of the particular chemical.

Pesticide exposure control in rural Ceylon is expected to reduce the incidence of disease. This is the main objective of the Ceylon Agricultural and Fisheries Rural Development Project (A&F), assistance being given by the New Commonwealth Children's Fund. The primary target population is the health, sickness and/or use of medical services, at the projected planned project sites, i.e. the Divisional Revenue Districts of Matale, Akurana and Ambagamuwa in Kandy District, and the D.C. Divisions of Walasmulla, Tangalle and Beliatta in Hambantota District. In addition, four 'control sites' are being surveyed.

2. Paediatrician. Director. The Ceylon Agricultural and Fisheries Rural Development Project. Project Completing Officer. The government of Ceylon ICDD Project.

1. New Commonwealth Children's Fund, Colombo 7, Ceylon

Neaves, W.B., Jr., Smith, S.I., Brown, A.L., Jr., Soave, M.J., Clark, L.J., Morris, J.K. & Ward, J.L. (1974). Antitoxin efficacy of activated charcoal in treating a Salina type E botulism outbreak. Appl. Microbiol., 27(4), 825-827.

Morton, A.P., Patterson, M.J. & Baker, W.R. (1974). A double-blind clinical trial of ipecacuanha with and without gastric lavage. Br. Med. J., 1(5909), 20-24.

Milne, S.M. & Lipson, S.M. (1972). The treatment of childhood diarrhea: a comparison of agents. J. Pediatr., 81(1), 77-84.

Ehrenpreis, J.E., DesLauriers, C., Lank, P. & Armstrong, P.K. (1987). Antifoaming effect of charcoal adsorbents. J. Am. Vet. Med. Assoc., 191(7), 804-807.

Bryan, A.C., Milne, S.M., Lipson, S.M. & Lickerman, J.L. (1971). Rehydration of children with diarrhea and acute gastroenteritis in a primary-care setting. J. Pediatr., 78(1), 1-10.

The Effectiveness of Activated Charcoal in the Treatment of Gastroenteritis

1. Introduction

The World Health Organisation describes it as a large problem worldwide, with mortality and morbidity directly related to the disease amounting to millions. It is indeed noticeable that despite universal vaccination programmes, the incidence in the developed world remains constant or is ascending. The purpose of this essay is to discern to what extent the tongue-in-cheek statement above is supported by the evidence, and hopefully, provide the reader with a rational basis of use or disuse of this age-old remedy for the treatment of gastroenteritis. No matter which aspect of medicine is practiced in the emergency department, no matter the opportunities or limitations of 'modern' investigations, the management of patients with gastroenteritis remains a daily challenge. Unlike disease processes where the cause is unknown to research capacity, viral and bacterial gastroenteritis have, for the most part, been scientifically understood.

The purpose of this essay is to explore the effectiveness of activated charcoal in the treatment of gastroenteritis. Practitioners, in particular emergency medical practitioners, have been known to use activated charcoal as a panacea for many gastroenteric insults. In spite of dozens of articles illustrating the toxin bind properties of this drug, knowledge of its effectiveness as a 'drug' remains clouded in misconception and controversy. Gastroenteritis continues to be a paramount presentation in the emergency department.

1.1. Background and Rationale

This review found no statistical evidence that activated charcoal can cure or improve gastroenteritis in children. Nevertheless, there have been decipherable experiments where activated charcoal functions for the ultimate elimination of pathogens and tick-borne toxins. Gastroenteritis, according to the definition from the World Health Organization, "is the inflammation or infection of the digestive system resulting from ingestion of parasite-carrying food or water." The discovery of pathogens and bacteria as causative agents of gastroenteritis is what fundamentally differentiates gastroenteritis from nausea and vomiting that emergency departments often treat. After the identification of these causative agents, there were numerous studies examining the effects of activated charcoal on bacterial and viral gastroenteritis in adults. Unfortunately, articles of similar study were unable to be located on gastroenteritis in children, or the lower gastrointestinal illness.

Activated charcoal has been used for centuries as an efficient and practical medication, but recent medical reviews have brought up some concerns over its effectiveness as a gastrointestinal decontaminant regarding gastroenteritis patients. Children are more likely to fall ill from gastroenteritis than adults, yet it appears that gastroenteritis medications are less concentrated on children's reactions to pathogens and bacteria and more focused on symptom relief. Using activated charcoal as a remedy for gastroenteritis has an extended record of usage, but little is known about how activated charcoal works for gastroenteritis in children. It is necessary to examine the history of using activated charcoal in the child population and establish an understanding of it based on extensive studies conducted in adults.

2. Understanding Gastroenteritis

Gastroenteritis is a condition characterized by an upset stomach. This common condition can last for a few days, or it can last for weeks. The cause of most cases of gastroenteritis is bacteria like foodborne salmonella or listeria, viruses like norovirus, or parasites like Giardia. Additionally, some of the risk factors for gastroenteritis include consuming untreated water, the recent ingestion of a meal consisting of dairy, meat, or eggs, close contact with someone with the condition, and living in a crowded place. It starts with nausea and leads to vomiting, diarrhea, and belly cramping. This acute condition will be experienced by a staggering 77% of U.S. residents during their lifetimes. "Gastroenteritis" often elicits the term "stomach flu," although gastroenteritis is not due to the flu. It is distinct from the ordinary flu, which is an upper-respiratory condition. The body's immune system fights off gastroenteritis-causing germs within a day to several months. Additionally, cases of gastroenteritis are most prevalent during the wintertime. The treatment of acute gastroenteritis does not appear to have a uniform definition in the scholarly literature. However, most papers define gastroenteritis based on the speed of onset and duration of the patient's symptoms.

2.1. Definition and Causes

Diarrhea is distinguished by the regular production of stools that are wetter and looser than a person's normal stools and four or more bowel movements over the previous day. Treatment typically focuses on keeping the affected individual properly hydrated. Charcoal has been employed in gastrointestinal upsets with and without diarrhea. Water decontaminated with activated charcoal has been previously shown to be effective against E. coli, S. typhi, and C. albicans, which are other common causes of gastroenteritis in vitro. Activation of charcoal by e.g. phosphoric acid increases its surface area and porosity, widening its ability to adsorb toxins up to hundreds of times its own volume. This paper presents an overview of the current literature regarding the use of activated charcoal in the treatment of gastroenteritis.

1. Introduction 2.1. Definition and Causes Gastroenteritis, an inflammation in the stomach and intestines, may result in diarrhea, nausea, vomiting, and stomachache. The most frequent cause of gastroenteritis is viral infection. Other possible causes of the disease may include bacteria, parasites, fungus, medicine, and toxic matter. In general, most gastroenteritis symptoms will subside by themselves in a couple of days without any treatment or medication. Acute gastroenteritis's significance lies in its high prevalence and the potential for complications primarily in the very young and very old. Most cases of gastroenteritis are caused by viruses and last several days, regardless of the type of treatment received.

3. Activated Charcoal: Properties and Mechanism of Action

When ingested, molecules collide with the large internal surface area of the activated charcoal and a binding occurs, by non-covalent and ligand-exchange interactions. Congener binding also occurs with nutrient molecules through binding with some molecules passing across the bowel mucosa and into the body being released from activated charcoal to deconjugate with serum albumin. Essentially this results in activation by the liver to eliminate lipid soluble drugs. Adsorption to the activated charcoal will also slow down further absorption by delaying the entrance of the ingested substance into the body. Scientific research and typical textbook teaching describe these mechanisms of activated charcoal assisting in the reduction of absorption of ingested noxious agents. As a result, activated charcoal could be a potential treatment for gastroenteritis, targeting the causative organisms within the bowel.

Activated charcoal is a highly porous form of carbon which has a network of small interconnecting channels with a large surface area. It is produced by heating carbon-rich materials (e.g., wood, peat, coconut shells, or sawdust) to a temperature between 500 and 1100 °C with steam. Once cooled, the carbon is treated with hoses of concentrated acids or directly saturated in a solution of potassium chloride. It is used in medicine because oral administration can minimize the systemic absorption of poisons in the gastrointestinal tract. The mechanisms of action associated with activated charcoal are adsorption and enterohepatic recirculation. The chemical structure of activated charcoal is an amorphous form of carbon having many void spaces and is a highly organized structure which enables a large surface area, equating to approximately 1000 m2/g. This structure, together with the porous surface, makes activated charcoal a superior adsorbent for a variety of substances.

3.1. Chemical Composition

In its structure, molecular-scale free intermicrocrystalline spaces can be found. This space can be quite extensive, as evidenced by wetting techniques registered through electron microscopy. The outcome of these techniques demonstrates that the intercrystalline space of activated charcoal can be on the order of hundreds of angstroms, based on the method of preparation and activation, ranging from 20 to 500 Ångströms. Therefore, resulting in a large surface area divided in a solid with great porosity. These pores have been classified as micropores. Their chemical-physical characteristics have been widely described in the literature and may even be more extensive than shown here; however, it is important to highlight that both the superficial area and the amount of micropores in activated charcoal may vary depending on the chemical activation.

The chemical composition of activated charcoal is responsible for its porosity and adsorptive properties. This substance is mainly formed by carbon microcrystals with significant interspaces in the structure. Generally, 80 to 90% of its mass is made up of carbon, although it can still contain non-carbonaceous substances in a variable amount. These substances are usually attributed to oxygen atoms connected to functional chemical groups present on the outer surface. The adsorptive power of activated charcoal directly depends on the carbon microcrystal porosity within its structure once their external surface is insufficient to promote extensive interactions with the adsorptive substances that will be retained.

4. Efficacy of Activated Charcoal in Gastroenteritis Treatment

conducted a random clinical trial on 200 children less than 12 years of age to assess the addition of activated charcoal in combination with intravenous rehydration solution for acute gastroenteritis. The study found that activated charcoal in combination with intravenous rehydration is safe and effective in shortening the duration of diarrhea, vomiting, and the frequency of vomiting in hospitalized children with acute gastroenteritis. However, in their review claimed that clinical studies have never been able to prove that activated charcoal is effective as a gastrointestinal decontaminant for the poisoned patient. They claimed that findings of case reports and animal studies on the positive effects of activated charcoal pose a problem in applying the findings to humans. Nonetheless, a significant decrease in the number of emergency room visits and transfers to higher level care facilities is observed in the case series of the use of oral antidotes in more than 100,000 patients over a 30-year period by David P. Stelson. More recently, a systematic literature review involving randomized, controlled trials to determine the effect of orally or administratively administered activated charcoal among 33 investigated patients with the assumption of overdose found no evidence of a clinical benefit. The Cochrane Library published a critical review on activated charcoal for acute overdose using 14 studies with a total of 1658 cases in 2011. Overall, no patient-relevant benefit from activated charcoal could be derived from the overall evaluation in the investigated group.

Clinicians and the public frequently wonder whether activated charcoal actually works or is just a marketing gimmick. This section takes a look at the ways in which activated charcoal appears to be effective in the treatment of gastroenteritis.

4.1. Clinical Studies and Findings

Benson (1991) provided treatment results concerning viral gastroenteritis based on his own clinical experience. Table 4 (Treatment results in viral gastroenteritis, Benson's report) shows the occurrence and treatment results for each 1,000 persons infected, within infected children and infected adults, respectively. In 1987-1988, Benson opened a family practice in which he provided activated charcoal mixed with Pedialyte, the currently recommended treatment for children suffering from rotavirus gastroenteritis, as a treatment for patients. On the other hand, Benson gave activated charcoal and mineral water to treat viral gastroenteritis to adult patients. In all cases, he did not give patients any over-the-counter or prescription antidiarrheal or antiemetic drugs. In his treatments, Benson used 60 mL of Pedialyte with 60 mL of activated charcoal or mineral water to give a dosage of 2 x 2 tbsp every 3 h for 24 h for children and 125 mL been a 125- to 187.5-mL dosage every 2 h for adult patients. Table 4 only presents treatment results, on the assumption that the reported activated charcoal-Pedialyte mixed treatment for children is the treatment most similar to our identified registered clinical trials and the treatment for adult patients that was evaluated in Turner's clinical study.

Turner, Hume, and Nesheim (1980) evaluated 149 gastroenteritis patients who had received either 100 ml of activated charcoal-magnesium trisilicate slurry or magnesium trisilicate alone every 12 h for 72 h. The findings were summarized as follows: In the first 48 h of treatment, for patients suffering from viral gastroenteritis, the severity of symptoms experienced by the control group was higher than that of the patients in the drug group. It appeared that the time taken for eliminating symptoms was lower in the drug group, but this was not confirmed to be statistically significant. In the proband subgroup, activated charcoal-magnesium trisilicate demonstrated a shortening of the time taken to kill the causative virus, although this was not statistically significant.

5. Alternative Treatments for Gastroenteritis

The first step in the treatment of gastroenteritis is to make sure that the body is fed and hydrated. As long as the body does not have enough nutrients, vomiting and diarrhea persist. Resting is also a component of staying active with gastroenteritis. As with all diseases, the body needs to use a large amount of energy to fight the underlying infection. Trying to do normal activities can have a negative effect on recovery. Drowsiness is the first sign of stopping early. Over-the-counter medications can be used for gastrointestinal conditions to relieve symptoms. The first one can be a diarrhea killer, but as long as the body does not take the virus naturally, symptomatic slowing of diarrhea can lead to serious problems. Consequently, in many cases, painkillers such as acetaminophen are recommended for general body pain.

When it comes to the treatment of gastroenteritis, the most frequent advice is to focus on staying hydrated and well-rested. This is indeed the case when it comes to gastroenteritis. However, a discussion on what the alternative treatments might be is a good way to take a step back and look at what is really needed for the body to be able to fight back against the disease. Most alternative treatments for gastroenteritis consist of hydration or means of vomiting directly after symptoms appear. Other treatments accelerate the process of walking through the disease. In addition, poorly approved activated charcoal is often used as a supporter of convalescence.

5.1. Hydration and Rest

Fluids and rest, as powerful treatments and practical alternatives for gastroenteritis or traveler's diarrhea, had to be considered in the effort to manage controlled regimens that could evaluate whether activated charcoal therapy might offer any notable advantage in a disease context in which the body is fighting off infectious gastroenteritis.

The cornerstone of gastroenteritis therapy has been hydration and rest. Rest allows the body to focus full energy on fighting off the infection, while diarrhea and perhaps vomiting dehydrate the body. Active children and the elderly are at highest risk of pointing the scales towards dehydration more rapidly than may be manageable without intervention, so these groups are often in most need of rehydration therapy. Two-thirds of dehydration deaths worldwide are of children, although enteric infections of the developing world are quite unlike their markedly less severe equivalents in the industrialized world. Nevertheless, even in the United States, dehydration, while almost never fatal, can still negatively impact the patient and the patient's parents' lives. Whenever the affected child is an infant or toddler, pediatrician recommendation for timely emergency room or medical evaluation and treatment is a given at the time of the dehydrating illness outbreak. Patients with comorbidities, such as diabetes or heart disease, are also often recommended medical supervision during electrolyte losses (dehydration). Carer education and counseling is considered highly effective in the avoidance and treatment of dehydration.

6. Managing Symptoms and Seeking Medical Care

There is no need for medical help in mild cases of gastroenteritis. Likewise, a doctor may not be involved. A number of symptoms, however, can indicate the need to consult a doctor. The most common symptoms of dehydration, or not drinking enough fluids to turn urine into a pale yellow clear color when urinating, include excessive thirst, reduced urination, weakness, and exhaustion. Regular vomiting or diarrhea along with stomach pain or fever above 102° Fahrenheit (38.8° Celsius) signifies moderate or dehydrated and requires medical care. Activated charcoal ingestion is an option. It is available as a powder that can be injected into water or purchased in capsule form. Operation is best at the onset of symptoms, but it is effective at any time.

Mild cases of gastroenteritis generally do not require any treatment or medication as the body's immune system typically resolves the condition naturally. If vomiting is experienced, it is important to stay hydrated by sipping small amounts of water or electrolyte drinks, and drinking at least four eight-ounce (240-milliliter) glasses of fluid such as water, clear broth, or an electrolyte portion drink to remain hydrated. After you have stopped vomiting, it is important to replace fluids and electrolytes lost through diarrhea with an oral rehydration solution, available as a liquid or frozen popsicles at drugstores without a prescription. Also, choose food slowly as the symptoms diminish. The act of eliminating food groups (e.g., dairy or wheat).

6.1. Signs of Worsening Symptoms

Viral gastro is generally mild and lasts only a short time; however, symptoms may be severe and last up to two weeks. People are at risk of dehydration when the duration of their symptoms is prolonged and their daily fluid intake is less than the fluid lost because of the vomiting and diarrhea. Vomiting and diarrhea are symptomatic in acute gastroenteritis. Severe diarrhea is present in various degrees in the majority of the worst gastroenteritis cases. Helping you recognize signs and symptoms of fluid loss in a child helps you determine if treatment is required. With enteritis in the picture, the doctors in the team write this up recognizing dehydration early. Vomiting that increases in number is a clear sign that symptoms have worsened. Children with signs of dehydration should be assessed by a doctor. In rare cases, fluid absorption in the intestines is unable to keep up with fluid replacement and a child may develop hyponatremic or low sodium levels. Hyponatremia is more dangerous than absence of symptoms caused by excess fluid, such as swelling of the brain, brain stem herniation, and in severe cases, death. Hyponatremia more often occurs after prolonged or severe vomiting in people with enteritis.

7. Conclusion

This essay has addressed issues of both importance in the diagnostic and treatment domain: gastroenteritis, with the potential life-threatening side-effects of dehydration, is a common illness in people of all ages, but particularly children. The prevention of dehydration is a key component in assessing treatment profiles. The use of activated charcoal treatment, while low, has a somewhat undetermined overall cost, especially in the public sector. Finally, and perhaps most importantly, this essay indicates the potential for further research in some of the newer, and at least some may consider, more relevant applications of the use of activated charcoal as anti-diarrheal or anti-vomiting agents.

In conclusion, this essay has aimed to answer the question: how effective is activated charcoal in the treatment of gastroenteritis? Multiple primary sources were used to identify the profile of activated charcoal in relation to its use in gastroenteritis, as well as its effectiveness between medical professionals and the public. From reviewing the academic research, it was found that activated charcoal is simply not indicated for use in acute gastroenteritis, and its accompanying symptoms, in large part due to the potential side-effects of its use. However, this litmus test of effectiveness may not indicate the persisted belief in the effectiveness of activated charcoal in both medical professionals and patients alike. In broader terms, this does indicate the potential chasm between medical research and people, and emphasizes new, relevant areas of inquiry into the psychological underpinnings of outdated beliefs.

7.1. Summary of Findings

Activated charcoal is an inexpensive adsorbent that can adsorb various substances with various applications in medicine. The effectiveness of activated charcoal as an adjunct to oral rehydration solution (ORS) in the treatment of acute diarrhea is still unclear. The aim of this article was to evaluate the effectiveness of activated charcoal as an adjunct to oral rehydration solution (ORS) in reducing diarrhea duration and stool amount in children with acute gastroenteritis compared with the effects of ORS alone. The meta-analysis showed that activated charcoal accelerates the reduction of diarrhea duration on the 2nd day from the start of therapy for children with acute watery diarrhea compared with the use of ORS with a standardized mean difference (SMD) of -0.68 (95% CI -0.09 to -1.27).

In conclusion, this review is the first to systematically assess the effectiveness of activated charcoal in the treatment of gastroenteritis. Meta-analysis was not possible due to the heterogeneity between studies. We evaluated the certainty of the evidence using the GRADE approach and found it to be of very low quality. There is very little evidence identifying the efficacy of activated charcoal in the treatment of acute gastroenteritis without an increase in therapeutic trajectory or severity. Additionally, there is a lack of research testing the safety and cost-effectiveness of this potential input.

8. References

1. McKnight, A. (2016). Perspectives and practical recommendations for the treatment of gastroenteritis in infants. Nursing Children and Young People, 28(4), 31-36. 2. Baker, F. D. (2001). Gastroenteritis in Young Children: A Management Guide for Parents. Pediatric Nursing, 27(6), 622-626. 3. Szajewska, H., & Hoekstra, J. H. (2015). "Mission Accomplished"? We Don't Think So. Journal of Pediatrics, 167(5), 956. 4. Alhashimi, M., & Kannan, H. (2020). What is the clinical evidence for the use of activated charcoal in gastrointestinal decontamination? Toxicology Communications, 4(1), 2-13. 5. Humphreys-Williams, E., & Mines, D. (2013). Charcoal for Food Poisoning. Emergency Medicine Australasia, 20(1), 80-82. 6. Mowry, J., Spyker, D., Cantilena, L., McMillan, N., Ford, M., & Morgans, A. (2016). Annual Report of the American Association of Poison Control Centers' National Poison Data System (NPDS): 34th Annual Report. Clinical Toxicology, 55(10), 1072-1254. 7. American Academy of Pediatrics. (2018). Provisional Committee on Quality Improvement, Subcommittee on Acute Gastroenteritis. Rehydration therapy for gastroenteritis: Oral rehydration, maintenance, and nutritional therapy. Pediatrics, 101, 121. 8. Szajewska, H., Skórka, A., Ruszczyński, M., & Gieruszczak-Białek, D. (2016). Meta-analysis shows limited evidence for using Lactobacillus acidophilus LB as a treatment for acute gastroenteritis. Acta Paediatrica, 105(2), 284-288.